REINVENTING REVENUE CYCLE MANAGEMENT:

DELIVERING NEXT-LEVEL PATIENT EXPERIENCES

REINVENTING REVENUE CYCLE MANAGEMENT:

DELIVERING NEXT-LEVEL PATIENT EXPERIENCES

By Marty Callahan, Casey Williams, and April Wilson

RevSpring Press (CreateSpace)

2018

Copyright © 2018 by Marty Callahan, Casey Williams, and April Wilson

All rights reserved. This book or any portion thereof may not be reproduced or used in any manner whatsoever without the express written permission of the publisher except for the use of brief quotations in a book review or scholarly journal.

First Printing: 2018

ISBN 9781982995706

RevSpring, Inc.
38705 Seven Mile Road, Suite 450
Livonia, MI 48152-3979
www.revspringinc.com

CONTENTS

Dedication vii

Chapter 1: The Power of Clear Communication 9

    Pre-Service Opportunities 11

    Point-of-Service Engagement 15

    After the Appointment 21

Chapter 2: Time is Critical 28

    The New Generation of Patients 28

    Your business office should never close 31

Chapter 3: When the Balance Shouts Over Your Words 36

    The 3 questions behind an effective statement design 37

    Making it "pretty" is good, but it's not enough 39

    Choosing the best file output for your SBO conversion (PDF vs. FTF) 41

Chapter 4: How They Pay Is Half the Battle 44

    Let Your Portal Do the Heavy Lifting 44

Chapter 5: Leverage Intelligence at Every Touchpoint 48

    Four steps to simplify account segmentation 48

    Want better results from predictive analytics? Try these proven strategies from other industries. 51

    Front-End vs. Back-End Scoring & Segmentation: Which is best for your health system? 53

Chapter 6: Ensure Compliance and Security 59

501(r): What You Need to Know 59
Is your healthcare organization ready for EMV? 64
What does it mean for healthcare providers? 65
Security Layers to Implement 66
Final Thoughts **67**
References **71**

Dedication

This book is for healthcare providers and partners who continue to have the courage to push the envelope and deliver world-class financial experiences to their patients. Thank you for the opportunities you have given us to study the patient experience in the never-ending quest for the best outcomes.

We'd also like to thank our contributing editors, Somlynn Rorie and Kate Leitao and our graphic design team, Christine Frandsen and Megan Ciaverelli.

MDLogic EHR → sends codes to charges

PM → so that we work as an all-in-one

EHR Documentation + Billing

Those codes/charges are provided → charges translate to codes/ in a claim alongside necessary documentation

+ then goes to the patient's insurance (payer [commercial or medicare])

Client does (when we expand this further)

Since MDLogic is handy this for clients rather than billing (copay) — we secure a percentage from those charges.

Ready elements operate as an all-in-one
EHR
PM
RCM

Chapter 1: The Power of Clear Communication

Patient communication is a critical component when it comes to clinical care, but it is equally important to the patient financial experience. Healthcare providers have three clear opportunities to educate, empower, and engage patients: pre-service, point-of-service, and post-service financial communications.

In an ideal world, revenue cycle management (RCM) facilitates patient payments seamlessly and promptly. However, in the real world, RCM requires much more than presenting a patient with a bill and then collecting a payment. Twenty years ago, it was perfectly acceptable to mail required patient statements since most payments came from payers—this is no longer our reality.

A crucial goal for RCM is to enhance the patient's financial experience, which leverages all available touchpoints for patient engagement and quickly expedites payment and account resolution. From an RCM perspective, an effective patient engagement strategy includes a laser-focus mindset on transforming traditionally underutilized consumer touchpoints to ensure an optimal financial outcome.

The healthcare industry would do well to follow and implement best practices taken from the most successful Business to Consumer (B2C) companies—regardless of sector. These companies have done the leg work, have become adept, and are successful at engaging customers at every step of the consumer purchasing journey. Such companies have set the stage for understanding and creating a satisfying customer experience throughout the buying cycle. By following their precedence, these best practices lead to higher payment, conversion rates, and customer loyalty.

Standard operating procedures for many B2C enterprises is to establish multiple digital touchpoints based on consumer behavior habits and to engage consumers before they visit the company's e-commerce site or brick-and-mortar store.

In Accenture's analysis in "Patient Loyalty: It's up for Grabs," research confirmed the correlation between a patient service experience, financial experience, and a patient's loyalty.[i] Patients are also consumers, and a patient/consumer wants and expects responsiveness and convenience when engaging in any payment experience.

Percent of consumers who indicated they would switch providers for...

47%
the ability to understand cost upon scheduling and to easily understand and pay a billing using a perferred method.

51%
great customer service

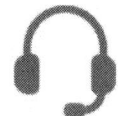

52%
the ability to get an appointment at a convenient location

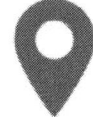

61%
the ability to get an appointment quickly when needed

Source: 2014 Consumer Health Study

In the following sections, we will examine how companies in the B2C space are using various communication touchpoints, which could be leveraged and used by healthcare providers to enhance the patient financial voyage.

Pre-Service Opportunities

For healthcare organizations, the revenue cycle begins with the patient's first contact with staff. A pre-service interaction includes appointment scheduling and eligibility verification. Pre-service is a neglected area and a missed opportunity that allows healthcare organizations to strengthen patient engagement by providing user-friendly tools, such as a pre-registration online portal and appointment reminders. Such tools utilize the patient's preferred communication channels and create a consumer/patient journey that they are accustomed to receiving.

Approaching appointment reminders differently

Because patients are now choosing their healthcare experience based on price, reviews from online media websites, and an organization's reputation for care, patient communications have gone from a nice-to-have to a must-have feature for any medical practice. With this significant shift toward value-based care, it isn't enough to just send messages and notifications. To make your patient experience most effective, healthcare organizations must prioritize the practice of sending the right messages, through the right channels, at the right time.

This section explores key attributes needed to successfully build an effective appointment reminder strategy.

Collecting Contact Preferences

The best way to reach your patients is to give them multiple communication options, which include notifications by phone, text, email, and online portal. The more contact options an organization offers to a patient, the higher the response rate.

Patients who only provide a phone number have the lowest response rate with just one in four outbound phone messages getting a reply.[ii] However, when a patient also provides an email and a cell number to text, the response rate jumps significantly. Adding text messages as an option has the most significant impact on patient response rates, increasing replies from one to three. When patients download an appointment reminder app, the response rates are even higher.

Omnichannel Communication

If your organization has four different options for contacting a patient, it does not mean a patient wants four different reminders, especially all at the same time.

A best practice to keep in mind is to send one reminder at a time, starting several days before the appointment. When the patient responds to confirm their attendance, other modes of communication should stop, and no other reminders should be sent. Start the message chain using a reminder app two weeks prior to the patient appointment and then send email reminders three days before the appointment, text messages two days before, and add a phone call the day before to maximize your pre-service communication strategy.

Recommended Settings:

App: 2 weeks prior to appointment
Email: 3-5 days prior to appointment
Text: 2 days prior to appointment
Call: 1 day prior to appointment

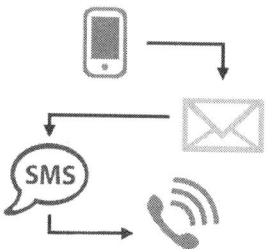

A Patient Preference Approach

Strive to make your omnichannel communication strategy tailored to the patient's needs by asking for their preferred contact mode. Don't just offer them one option—offer multiple modes, such as a call, text, and email and let them choose which communication model works best for their needs.

Patient Information	Contact Information		Patient Preference
Name: Jane Doe	Home Phone: 555-123-4567		Text [X] [ ]
Patient No: 12345	Cell Phone: 555-987-6543		Email [X] [ ]
DOB: 1/2/1934	Email: janedoe@example.com		Call [ ] [X]

12

The Weight of a Phone Call

Many patients still prefer receiving a phone call reminder instead of a text message or email. Research on this topic indicates that patients prefer call reminders to be short and sweet. Keep your call scripts simple and to the point. Patients tend to stop listening after around 45 seconds.

> *"Hello, this is Main Street Medical calling to remind you of your upcoming appointment at our West Office with Dr. Smith. The appointment is for John on Tuesday, July 15th, at 2:00 p.m. To confirm the appointment, press 1. If you need to reschedule, press 2. Thanks and we look forward to seeing you."*

Timing is Everything

Different modes of communication have different approaches to that drive optimize response. Phone call response rates, for example, increases at certain times of the day. Studies have found patients are most responsive to phone calls at 4:00 p.m, as well as 5:00 p.m, 3:00 p.m., and 9:00 a.m. Calling during lunch hours is the least likely time to get a response or answer.

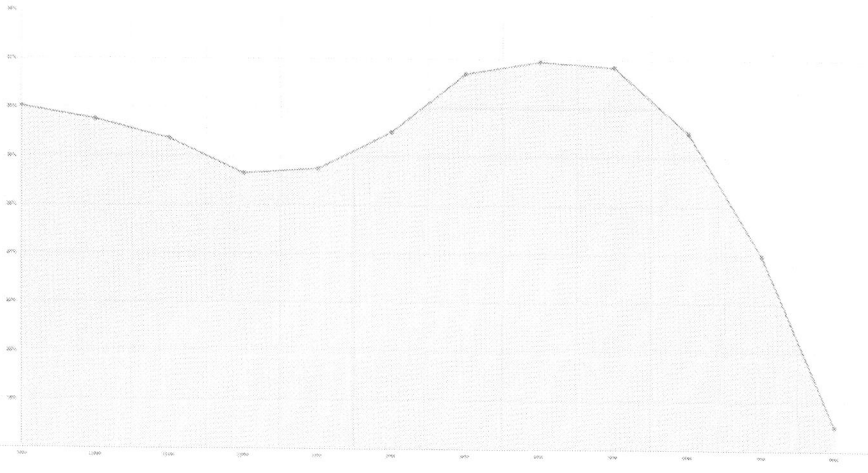

OPTIMIZING TIMING
Patients are most responsive at **9 am and between 3pm - 5pm.**

The Length of a Text Message

Text messages are limited to 160 characters, so maximize each word when creating your automated text program. This is especially critical since consumers tend to check their phones an average of 80 times per day.[iii] Some smartphones will automatically create clickable links from texts (including address and phone number), so be sure to test across different devices.

> Jane, you have an appointment with Main Street Medical on August 15 at 3:30 p.m. Reply CONFIRM or RESCHED. Questions? 555-123-4567

> Confirm

Point-of-Service Engagement

Ideally, frontline staff is equipped with innovative, best-in-class, RCM technology that can tailor patient engagement and impact a positive financial outcome. This technology offers built-in functionality for estimating patient balances, segmenting financial risk, automating payment arrangements, and accepting payments during a patient's point-of-service.

A point-of-service collection initiative should already be in place within your organization that includes the proper tools, technology, and staff training. If you've already implemented a sound patient engagement strategy on the front end (one that influences more patients to pay at the point-of-service), what's next?

How do you motivate and influence your registrar staff to keep improving? How do you keep moving the needle on your point-of-service collection efforts?

Conventional wisdom (and common sense) provides managers and supervisors with basic guidelines for enhancing point-of-service objectives. Setting goals, giving praise, offering incentives, and communicating results and performance are all important components to keep the momentum going. Yet, research also has suggested that how you execute these tasks can make a tremendous difference in your staff's performance.

Here are three simple adjustments managers can make to boost their team's performance – and ultimately their point-of-service collections.

1. Don't set overly specific goals

When it comes to setting goals, whether for ourselves or others, we often end up being very specific. In our personal lives, we create goals such as exercising 30 minutes a day, getting seven hours of sleep each night, or losing two pounds a week. Collection goals set for registrar teams may be similarly specific—collect a specific dollar amount per month or increase overall point-of-service collections by a certain percentage over last month's rate.

However, research has found this may not be the best approach. **Instead of setting specific number goals, studies have indicated setting a high-low goal range can lead to better results.** For example, instead of setting a monthly collection increase goal of three percent, a more optimal approach would be to set a high-low range approach, such as setting a goal for a two to four percent increase in point-of-service collections.

Research published by Harvard researchers[iv] found a high-low goal approach is more effective because it satisfies two key factors that drive people to achieve a goal—challenge and attainability. This means for a goal to be effective, it must be perceived as sufficiently challenging (which ultimately feeds a personal sense of accomplishment) and must also be viewed as realistically attainable to prevent people from abandoning their attempts of achieving it.

The high-low goal range approach is especially applicable in a team setting, in which there is a mix of low, medium, and high performers. **A high-low goal range allows managers to challenge high** performers without making performance targets feel unattainable to lower performers.

2. Focus on Incremental Progress

Consistent, internal communications that communicate progress and performance of the high-low goal help managers encourage their staff, boost morale, and creates an obtainable objective for staff. But, more importantly, it is the context in which progress is communicated that can influence the motivation levels of team members.

What is known as the "small-area hypothesis[v]," studies have suggested that when a person's focus is set on smaller amounts of progress made or efforts remaining, people are more encouraged to accomplish tasks and meet goals.

For internal communications, focus on the small amount of progress that has already been made by your team. Then, after the team has crossed the halfway mark, focus on the smaller amount of effort that is remaining to complete the goal.

Take for example, your LinkedIn profile—the networking site prompts you to complete your online profile with a message like:

You are **20% away from completing** your online profile:

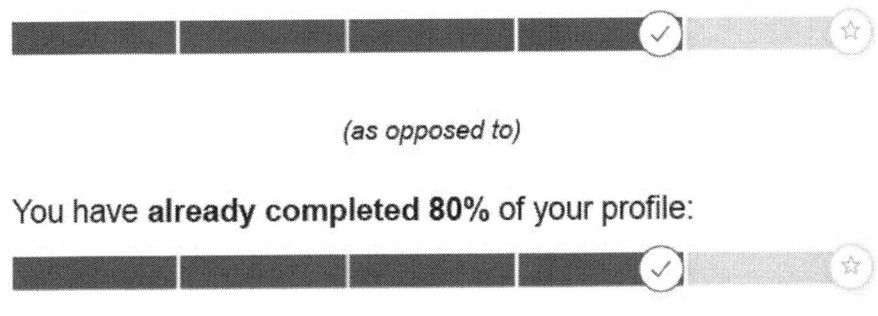

(as opposed to)

You have **already completed 80%** of your profile:

Both messages are true; but, instead of focusing attention to the larger number, LinkedIn directs your focus to the smaller amount of effort remaining – hoping to increase your motivation to complete your online profile.

On the other end of the spectrum, in the early stages of accomplishing a task or goal, it is better to focus on the small amount of progress that has been made. For example, if your team has a monthly collection goal and had a great first week of the month, it's better to communicate:

We're only one week in and you've **already collected 35%** of your monthly target!

(...instead of)

We've made a great start to this month, and only have **65% of the way to go**...

The change is subtle, but it may be the difference in getting your staff to remain committed to the goals you set.

3. Use Incentives Wisely

While there's no denying the power of incentives to sway human behavior, research in consumer behavior suggested that we often miss the mark when we offer incentives to improve motivation and performance.

What studies[vi] have found is that we wrongfully assume the people we are trying to influence will automatically see the advantage of our offer.

For example, if a manager offers a $25 gift card to each team member that meets his or her collection goal, we expect those team members to understand the value of the offer. However, this is not necessarily the case, and there is the risk that incentives like this can be perceived as something the employee is entitled to simply for doing their job as opposed to demonstrating excellent behavior.

Studies have also shown[vii] that incentives are more effective at influencing behavior when the offer itself is accompanied with the advantages of the offer. If a manager is offering her staff a $25 gift card, she may also want to ask them to think about how they would spend the $25 gift card. What would they buy? If it's a gift card for a restaurant, what meal would they plan on ordering? If the incentive is a paid vacation day, what would they spend their day off doing?

These insights do not suggest managers and supervisors should completely abandon current point-of-service collection processes and employee incentives but to approach and utilize them in a more mindful way.

4. Make Results Transparent

However you choose to structure your incentive program, make sure that everyone can see how their performance is tracking against your goals. You can do this digitally via an automated dashboard as part of your standard customer service interface, or you can do it "old-school" with a bulletin board tracking progress in common areas. It is critical to be transparent with progress to avoid the potential risk of personal bias and even the playing field.

5. Leveraging predictive analytics

In today's crowded healthcare marketplace, hospitals and providers, already facing dwindling reimbursements, must adopt new strategies to accelerate revenues, reduce bad debt, and make it easier for patients to pay. From a revenue cycle perspective, deploying innovative technologies that leverage the power of healthcare technologies to enhance performance is a business imperative. Such technologies include data analytics, which provide critical insight into the effectiveness of an organization's revenue cycle workflows.

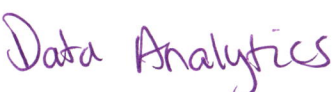
Data Analytics

By taking advantage of data analytics, hospitals and providers can gain a better understanding of patient payment behaviors, as well as identify causes for the rejection of claims and determine the effectiveness of their collection efforts.

Data analytics have helped to transform healthcare delivery and revenue cycle management by making it possible for facilities to organize and manage large volumes of clinical and financial data. Since more hospitals and providers have turned to data analytics to improve revenue cycle processes, tracking key metrics (such as clinical results, account consolidations, and claims tracking) across the organization has become easier and more streamlined. Data analytics become even more important for healthcare organizations in the era of value-based reimbursement models, in which quality measures must be reported to receive the highest possible reimbursement from payers.

A key benefit of data analytics is that hospitals and providers can evaluate and benchmark the information being collected. This enables healthcare organizations to determine which data measurements are mission-critical for enhancing the revenue cycle. Data reports can isolate important trends that have an impact on revenues. From clinical data to payment information, data analytics provide hospitals and providers with a complete picture of revenue cycle workflows. When healthcare organizations take advantage of available analytics technology to pinpoint specific deficiencies in the revenue cycle, workflows can be optimized to achieve better results.

Data analytics also help with decisions about cost containment and cash flow. With data analytics integrated into the revenue cycle workflow, hospitals and providers can learn more about the propensity-to-pay of specific patient demographics and why some claims are rejected by insurance companies. The insights gleaned from reports can be used by healthcare organizations to enhance patient engagement and reduce denials, which contributes to greater cash flows.

From gaining an understanding of patient payment behaviors to identifying which revenue cycle processes require tweaking, there's no question that healthcare organizations stand to benefit greatly from the use of data analytics. To keep up with the ever-changing landscape of healthcare delivery, hospitals and providers can leverage data analytics to ensure that no healthcare dollars are left on the table while delivering a positive patient experience.

After the Appointment

Healthcare organizations are walking a fine line between providing high-quality, affordable medical care and protecting revenues to ensure their own financial health. The changing landscape of reimbursement, driven by new value-based payment models and greater financial responsibility being passed on to patients, has placed hospitals and providers in a must-act position: Revamp legacy revenue cycle processes or potentially watch money go out the door.

Post-discharge and follow-up initiatives can increase the financial performance in multiple ways. The transmission of targeted, patient-specific messages using the consumer's preferred communication channels can be optimized to deliver a personalized patient experience that can facilitate quicker payment.

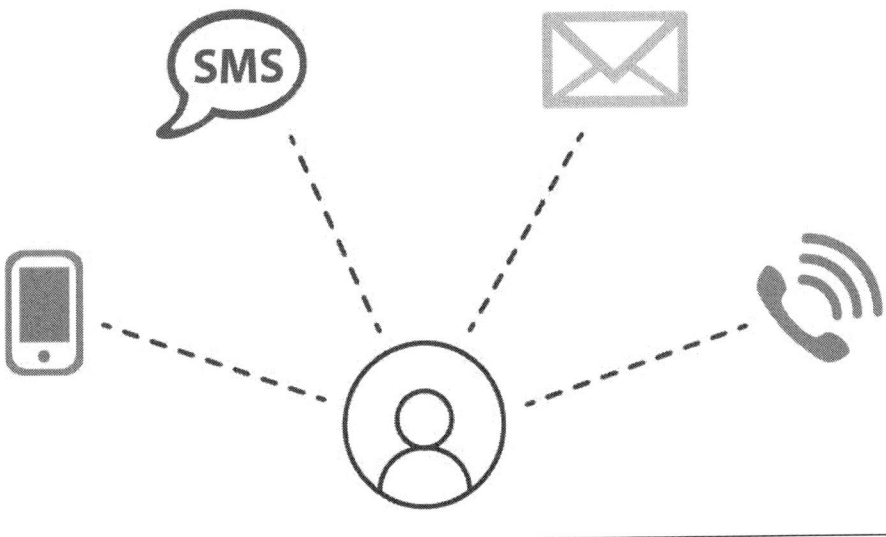

Post-discharge and follow-up patient engagement also provides a viable opportunity for revenue collection. A robust and scalable RCM technology solution integrated with a highly automated engagement platform allows organizations to streamline the delivery of adherence messaging, patient satisfaction surveys, feedback reporting, and benchmarking. These follow up messages are an opportunity not to just get feedback survey but to gently prepare the patient and make the payment obligations more palatable.

Enhance Patient Satisfaction on the Financial Side

Today's empowered consumers expect tailored experiences and nearly half would switch providers to have greater healthcare financial transparency and higher service quality, according to TK[viii]. Patient satisfaction is not just limited to clinical care. Leaders of revenue cycle departments must recognize that the financial side of healthcare is also part of the overall patient experience.

How financial information is presented in a billing statement can make the difference between a satisfied patient and a dissatisfied one. More healthcare organizations are assessing their billing statements and opting to redesign them to improve patient satisfaction. RevSpring's proprietary focus group results have indicated that the more complicated and hard-to-understand a billing statement is, the more likely it is to go unpaid.

Well-designed, itemized statements that explain how much is owed and why, as well as clear instructions for submitting payments, boost patient satisfaction and the probability of the bill being paid. Satisfied patients are loyal and can provide a much-needed recurring revenue stream for hospitals and providers.

Make Your Self-Pay Communications Personal

Self-pay patients represent a real financial challenge for hospitals and providers. The non-profit Kaiser Family Foundation[ix] conducted a survey that revealed 20% of working families with health insurance struggle to pay their medical bills. Not surprisingly, the number was even higher for the uninsured population, with more than 50% stating they could not afford to pay for healthcare services received. When patients don't pay, the revenue cycle slows, cash flow shrinks, and bad debt grows. Healthcare organizations can get ahead of this issue by engaging patients at all stages of the revenue cycle.

There are multiple touchpoints where hospitals and providers should provide clear and effective communication to patients regarding their financial responsibility. Reaching out to patients regarding financial matters using targeted, personalized messaging is an important component of an effective patient engagement strategy. To reach a positive financial outcome, hospitals and providers must tailor patient communications at every stage of engagement through the channels each patient prefers. Channels should include phone, email, mail, and text message.

Make It Easy for Patients to Pay

From balancing a bank account to paying a mortgage, consumers are accustomed to managing their financial affairs electronically. Health organizations are making it easier for patients to review and pay their accounts by deploying self-service tools, like online patient portals. These tools enable hospitals and providers to respond to patients' expectations for private, quick, and convenient payment methods, which can ultimately shorten the revenue cycle.

Other options for self-pay include interactive voice recording (IVR) calls and mobile payment apps. The timely delivery of email and text-based statements, which contain a link to an online payment portal can also streamline bill payments. These self-pay tools remove obstacles and provide patients with the freedom to settle accounts at their convenience—which enhances their financial experience.

Additionally, using a superior RCM solution that leverages data analytics and predictive scoring to access the patient's propensity to pay, allows healthcare organizations to offer flexible payment options that increase their chances of getting paid and reduce costs associated with protracted collection efforts.

Statement design matters

Since the launch of the Healthcare Financial Management Administration's (HMFA) "Patient Friendly Billing Project" in 2000, the healthcare industry has made a concerted effort to improve patient billing practices. But there are still improvements to be made. According to a 2016 Mad*Pow patient billing survey[x], six in ten patients described medical bills they received as "confusing" or "very confusing." This means that 60 percent of the patients surveyed had no idea which medical services were being billed on their statements. With more patients making larger out-of-pocket payments for their healthcare, hospitals and providers must address the issue of poorly designed billing statements. Neglecting to do so could lead healthcare organizations down a perilous path toward bad debt and patient dissatisfaction.

A one-size-fits-all approach yields poor results

Every healthcare organization is a distinct entity, as are the communities they serve. For this reason, a one-size-fits-all approach to statement design is likely to yield poor results. To increase the success of their self-pay collection efforts, hospitals and providers must abandon the cookie-cutter formula for statement design in favor of intelligent statement design. The overarching objective of intelligent statements is to eliminate patient confusion by providing clear and concise account information, which can increase the likelihood of balances being paid on time. The key advantages and appeal of the intelligent statement are its simple design, omission of jargon, and overly technical language. Equally as important, an intelligent statement is personalized to the patient's unique financial profile, which typically uses meaningful data such as payment propensity scores to help determine the patient's financial profile.

The ability to group patients into segments based on past financial behavior (also known as predictive segmentation) enables healthcare organizations to be proactive in generating targeted communications that will elicit the desired patient response, i.e. prompt bill payment. In this kind of scenario, patients with a high propensity-to-pay score are segmented into one group, while patients with lower payment ratings are separated into another group. By utilizing predictive analytics and patient segmentation, hospitals and providers can personalize the billing statement experience based on an individual patient's unique financial and payment history.

HIGH	MEDIUM	LOW	CHARITY
More than $25	More than $500	More than $25	
	$25 - $500		
	LESS THAN $25		

An effective patient collection strategy entails much more than simply generating a statement and waiting for the dollars to roll in. According to the global management consulting firm, McKinsey & Company, hospitals and providers can expect to collect just 50 to 70 percent on balance-after-insurance (BAI) accounts[xi]. Conversely, other industry surveys have found that 90 percent of patients are likely to pay before the physician encounter, and another 70 percent will pay at checkout[xii]. Considering these figures, it has become critical for healthcare organizations to review their current revenue cycle technologies and workflows to ensure they are effectively engaging self-pay patients—or risk leaving money on the table.

The use of powerful and sophisticated health information technology for improving clinical outcomes, as well as financial performance has become ubiquitous across healthcare. Many healthcare organizations are wisely choosing to partner with an experienced RCM vendor to deploy the right mix of technology, workflows, and patient engagement strategies to help maximize collections and shorten collection times. One of the most impactful financial trends in healthcare has been the implementation of an end-to-end RCM solution that utilizes data analytics that gives providers actionable insight into a patient's propensity to pay. In the all-important area of self-pay accounts, best-in-class RCM technology coupled with the right patient engagement strategy can help organizations realize increases in three critical areas of self-pay: collected balances at first statement, self-service payments, and payment-in-full via interactive voice response (IVR) systems.

Increase Collected Balances at First Statement

It is difficult to collect balances from patients once they have left a medical office. RCM best practices suggest that patients should be engaged in the first 30 days post-service, when the probability of collecting some form of payment is higher, and the costs are lower to do so.

Increase Self-Service Payments Online

Healthcare consumers have vocalized that they expect their healthcare providers to offer access to self-service payment options. Hospitals and providers must accommodate today's digitally savvy patient by providing self-service technology that gives them a measure of control over their own healthcare experiences.

Technology tools that let patients privately, quickly, and conveniently manage both their clinical and financial matters can improve overall patient satisfaction. Healthcare organizations that take advantage of RCM technology that lets patients make payments anytime or anywhere, such as through an online portal, smartphone, or IVR system, generally realize an increase in self-service payments.

Payments in Full Using IVR

IVR is a secure and cost-effective way to enhance patient collec IVR technology enables hospitals and providers to receive payme 24/7 without the assistance of a live operator. The deployment of a PCI DSS-compliant IVR system will give patients the control they want, when they can make a payment, and how much they will pay. More importantly, IVR makes it possible for healthcare organizations to collect on accounts more quickly while increasing customer satisfaction.

Other benefits of an IVR include reduced inbound call volumes, lower call abandonment rates, and shorter wait times.

To remain financially viable, healthcare organizations must look beyond traditional approaches to revenue cycle management. By utilizing technology to focus on these three key financial metrics, hospitals and providers can capture more dollars from their self-pay patients.

Chapter 2: Time is Critical

The New Generation of Patients

With today's patients paying for a greater share of their healthcare costs, many are also paying closer attention to their providers' practices and policies—one group of patients rising to the forefront and are shaping the changing healthcare landscape are "Centennials."

Centennials constitute 25% of the U.S. population and are growing in number. Born between 1993 and 2017, this generation has already taken root in society—affecting buying trends, culture, social media, and political movements.

Healthcare organizations must take note: This generation has high expectations, though perhaps not as predictable as the "selfie" millennial patients. Centennials are largely driven by their values—one of the greatest being financial stewardship. They have lived through plummeting economies and fiscal instability. Centennial patients want to know that their hard-earned money will be used responsibly. For example, does your facility have a recycling policy? Have you invested in efficient, secure technology for both patient health records and payment processing? Do you make your budget and expenditures available to the public?

Financial transparency is only one piece of the equation in meeting centennials' expectations. Social justice is the heart of this generation, meaning charity care, public outreach programs, and community support play central roles in gaining their interest and trust. As they weigh their options for healthcare providers—and they certainly comparison-shop for doctors, urgent care services, and more—centennials take into consideration a health corporation's stance toward and treatment of the societal working class, impoverished, single-parent families, immigrants, and other key demographics.

Beyond financial and social implications, healthcare practices must take heed of this generation's knack for technology. Never has a generation been so reliant on technology. Their expectations of technology in the marketplace will drive their choices, perhaps even more than their finances. Starting with online reviews and ending with billing communications, centennials are tremendously deterred by outdated or uninformed technology across healthcare services.

Their ideal healthcare journey may look something like the following:

PATIENT JOURNEY

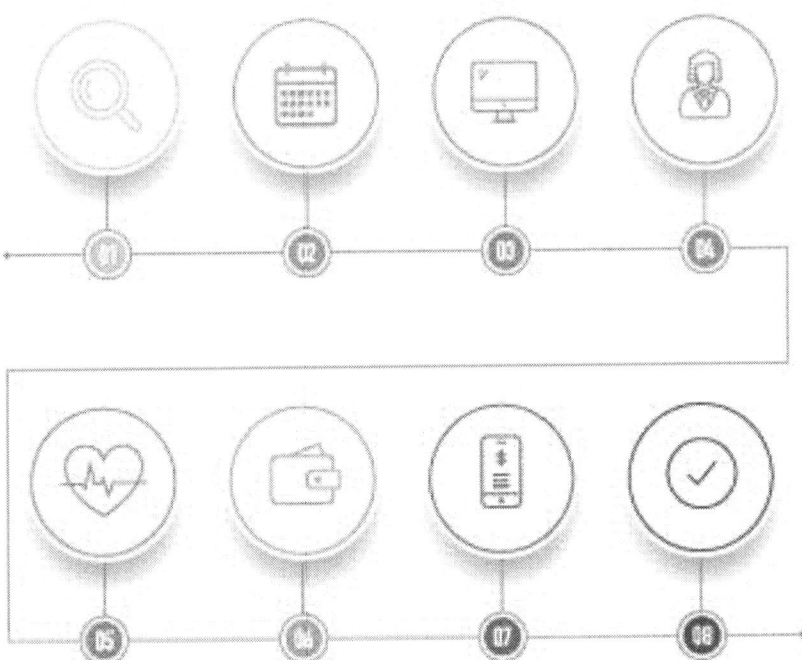

- Search for the right healthcare provider online in order to evaluate patient reviews, prices of services, and corporate practices
- If a virtual consultation isn't possible, schedule and register for an in-person appointment

- Check in online
- Be seen by the physician, who takes notes on a mobile device
- See that personal electronic health records are being updated in real time, including the option of syncing data from any wearable, health-monitoring technology
- If possible and sensible, pay upon exit
- Receive a clear, concise bill/receipt via the preferred method of communication (e.g. email or text) with itemized services, any fees owed, insurance coverage, and many convenient payment options
- Complete a succinct survey to inform the facility of how it can improve

While many of these tasks are in the hands of hospital boards and healthcare workers, a surprising amount falls into the realm of RCM. To secure revenue, RCM staff must understand today's patients and interact with them according to their preferences and needs. A cold, unexpected, or convoluted medical bill could have a negative impact that is large enough to keep a centennial from paying.

Thanks to this new generation, patient engagement is reaching new levels. Have you prepared?

Start With IVR

Patient engagement is not just about health facilities encouraging patients to make decisions about their healthcare. A successful patient engagement strategy also requires the deployment of cutting-edge technology tools that provide convenient and secure access to personal healthcare information, whether clinical or financial. To get patients to pay their bills, healthcare organizations are wisely leveraging technology, such as modern IVR systems.

Modern IVR systems offer automated outbound and inbound call functionality. An outbound IVR system can be programmed to contact patients when and where they are most likely to be reached. An inbound IVR provides flexible self-service payment options that enable patients to pay their medical bills without having to speak to a customer service agent unless they choose to do so.

More importantly, IVR gives patients the convenience and freedom of checking balances, making a single or recurring payment, or setting up a payment plan using a credit card, debit card, or automatic bank draft (ACH) any time during the day, 24/7/365.

Though the benefits of an IVR are many, not all IVR systems are created equal. To increase the likelihood of patient adoption, the IVR system must be convenient. The development of a truly intelligent IVR requires an understanding of human psychology and insight into the patients with whom the hospital or provider wishes to engage.

Data analytics such as communication preferences and propensity-to-pay scores, let healthcare organizations deploy an intelligent IVR system that will enable hospitals and providers to take advantage of captured data. This data can then be used to strengthen an organization's communications strategy and also provide valuable metrics, such as peak hours, the number of callers attempting to make a payment, the number of completed payments or unfinished payments, as well as other valuable data points. Additionally, a best-in-class intelligent IVR system will feature multi-language support, include customizable call routing, and ensure HIPAA and PCI DSS compliance.

More and more consumers are using their telephones (both cell phones and landlines) to handle their financial affairs, and they expect healthcare organizations to offer self-service, pay-by-phone payment options. The deployment of an intelligent IVR system will provide healthcare organizations with a return on investment in the form of accelerated revenues, reduced collection costs, and increased patient satisfaction.

Your business office should never close

Most hospitals and healthcare providers have internal initiatives that allow patients to set up online accounts to manage their health records and make payments for medical services. When patients pay via self-service, the average days from statement to payment is 14.3 and by phone it's 14.6. Compared to lockbox payments, which are 16 days on average from statement to payment, this can have significant impacts on time to cash for most health systems.

The greatest challenge is to increase patient comfort paying online or by phone, particularly among older patients. Americans age 65 and older make up about 15% of the population today, but by 2050 they will account for 22% of the population[xiii]. While this population is becoming more comfortable with new technology, 48% have reported that they need someone to help them learn how to use new technology such as smartphones, tablets, and laptops.[xiv]

That isn't to say that this group doesn't own technology, despite the challenges. About four in 10 older Americans own smartphones, up from 18% in 2013[xv]. About half of them have broadband in their homes, and 67% access the internet daily.

Older people are less likely to use self-serve

The strongest relationship between determining who will pay with self-service and any other factor is patient age. The graph on the next page illustrates this dynamic. It is important to note that this graph was purely descriptive, looking for key differences in the populations likely to leverage "traditional" payment methods like check by mail or customer service versus those likely to take advantage of digital self-service options like online portals and IVR. Research from this study/graph representation examined who is paying by payment channel and not why they chose those channels.

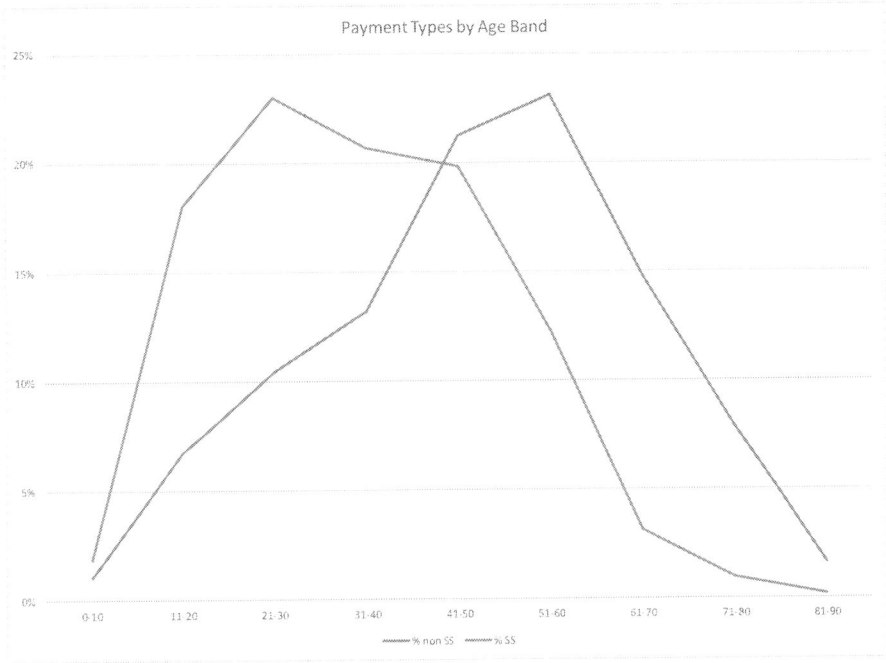

In the graph, the first line (% Self-Service) shows the age distribution of self-service payments while the second line shows the distribution of non-self-service payments (checks in the mail and customer service).

Drilling down into the detail of self-service payments, the age gap continues to widen when channel is considered. Younger payers are more likely to pay online, followed by inbound IVR.

The median age of someone paying via IVR is 47 years old, and the median age of someone paying online is 43 years old. While this doesn't suggest a huge age gap in likelihood to pay by IVR versus portal, when plotted by distribution, the differences in the populations become more pronounced. Most online portal payments fall into the 31 to 40 age group and most IVR payments fall into the 51 to 60 age band.

Implications for Healthcare Providers

To move the needle on encouraging older populations self-serve, several clear implications have emerged from industries outside of healthcare that should be adopted within healthcare:

1) Clearly communicate how to pay via self-serve on all patient communications. Your bill should offer the payment URL and language about how online payments are safe and secure to help build confidence in an older demographic.

2) Offer quick pay. While many hospitals and health systems have included this language on billing statements to help drive meaningful use, much of that language has been hyper-focused on requiring patient registration to set up a portal account before a patient can pay. Given that over 85% of online payments are "quick pay" (the ability to make a payment without account creation), you may be putting up barriers to online self-service if you require patient portal registration.

3) Offer educational videos about how to pay online or by phone. Waiting rooms are a unique opportunity to do patient education about healthcare management. Many healthcare providers have televisions in their waiting rooms but may not be making the most of having a captive audience waiting to be seen. It is an industry best practice to showcase community health initiatives, online website options, and the convenience of paying by phone 24/7/365. Younger demographics are probably looking at their phones, but older demographics will probably be watching the television. (Adults ages 65 and over watch television three times more than their younger counterparts.) An explainer video showing how easy and safe it is to pay online is a great feature to have displayed in the waiting room—leverage that same educational content on patient portals, as well.

4) Do not try to push people out of their comfort zones. If your target audience is younger, you may want to more prominently feature online payment as the top payment

option on all printed and digital payment communications. If your target audience is older, you may want to feature how to pay by phone. You'll be far more successful driving response in channels where certain demographics have their comfort levels already set.

Chapter 3: When the Balance Shouts Over Your Words

It's a known reality that patient payments continue to decrease in the face of escalating medical costs per individual.[xvi]

Age	Median Household Income	Average Bill Amount
15 - 24	$ 34,645	$ 807.33
25 - 34	$ 54,305	$ 929.46
35 - 44	$ 66,770	$ 803.33
45 - 54	$ 70,913	$ 789.08
55 - 64	$ 60,650	$ 752.39
65 +	$ 36,937	$ 276.14

TABLE ABOVE REFERENCES REVSPRING PROPRIETARY RESEARCH

The right patient statement design can be a remarkably powerful tool for healthcare business offices. Today's RCM leaders are recognizing this opportunity, and looking for ways to capitalize on what has traditionally been an underutilized touchpoint in the revenue cycle process.

And for most organizations, this means requesting patient statement design "best practices" in an RFP or in a conversation with their current vendor. Then, statement design samples are reviewed by the organization and they choose which design(s) they like best.

While this can be a good starting point, only focusing on proclaimed "best practices" or simply copying what another healthcare organization is doing has its limitations.

It's a matter of context. One organization's "best practices" may or may not work for a given situation. The most critical factor is

if the presented balance will overshadow anything else on your printed statement.

But there is a process that *does* always work. A process that, when done correctly, significantly impacts RCM performance – boosting cashflow, cutting AR days, reducing the cost to collect self-pay dollars.

In short, it's an efficient and scalable approach to engaging patients in the billing process with targeted messages - leading to better business outcomes for your revenue cycle.

The 3 questions behind an effective statement design

The most effective patient statement redesigns, and patient engagement strategies, start by answering these three questions.

Question #1: What do you know about your business and processes?

Start by asking, "What components of our revenue cycle and business office must we keep in mind during this process?"

This step is all about narrowing the focus of your patient engagement strategy. Really understanding the strengths and weaknesses of your current operations, so your communication design will fit the needs that are specific to your organization and billing environment.

You should account for things like:

- Resources
- Limitations (staff or technological-related)
- Technology
- Problem areas

The key here is to pay attention to the areas that cause –or have the potential to cause – friction or complexity for your patients during your current account resolution process.

Question #2: What do you know about your patient population?

After assessing the strengths and weaknesses of your current process, it's time to outline what you know about the patients you serve.

You should account for things like:

- The top reasons patients call your business office
- Past payment behavior (How soon do most patients pay? First Notice? Second Notice?)
- Current self-service adoption rate (Example: Online bill pay or IVR payment)

This a great time to leverage analytic intelligence, if your organization is using predictive scores to segment patient accounts.
Understanding a patient's ability and likelihood to pay, combined with current behavioral metrics, allows for a more targeted (and effective) communication strategy.

Question #3: What do you want your patients to do?

Now, based on what you know about your processes and your patient population – what do you want your patients to do?

This final component is what ultimately guides the statement design process. It's about creating a well-defined resolution funnel for the different scenarios your business office encounters.

Based on these scenarios, and the factors that keep patients from resolving their accounts, how do you leverage design and messaging to get patients to take the desired action?

Here are some of the common scenarios we see:

- For patients that can pay in full, how will you influence them to pay faster? Or pay using more cost-efficient self-service channels?
- For patients that can't pay in full, how do you influence them to take action, and get enrolled in a payment plan?
- For patients that qualify for financial assistance or charity care, how do you influence them to complete the proper paper work and avoid being placed in Bad Debt?

How precise these scenarios get will depend greatly on the current technologies you have in place, the business problems you face, the print capabilities of your communication solution provider, etc.

What is important to point out however, is that this process creates an environment to where each scenario has one specific goal – making it much easier to track and monitor the effectiveness of your patient communication strategy.

Making it "pretty" is good, but it's not enough
A visually appealing statement design has its merits.

Numerous research studies show that aesthetically attractive design has a major psychological influence on us humans. It builds trust, credibility, and is more likely to result in action being taken.

There's more to design than making something look pretty. Good design makes something functional, visually communicating importance to drive the optimal response. And you decide what is most important to communicate by going through the 3-step process outlined above.

This process gets even more complicated when you are preparing for an SBO conversion.

Here are some of the key challenges health systems should prepare for when designing or redesigning their SBO patient statement series – and some tips to improve their effectiveness.

Challenge #1: Connecting the balance to the occurrence and location

When physician and hospital charges are combined within the same communication, patients have difficulty understanding which balance correlates with which facility and occurrence.

First, using white space and dynamic color can help visually segment information and reduce patient confusion in any billing environment. This approach holds true in the SBO environment as well.

However, what is unique to SBO statements is the need to clarify charges *by location or facility*.

To make this connection, our clients utilize "icon-like" graphics, based on their data file. This approach makes it easy for patients to see how their charges break-down by service location.

Challenge #2: Clearly communicating the age of each balance

The amount of information presented to patients in an SBO bill can make it difficult to understand what they owe – or at least what they owe *now*. This is especially true in a communication that contains multiple occurrences.

The last thing a health system wants is for a patient to be placed in bad debt because he or she did not understand the timeline of their outstanding account(s).

To provide clarity to their patients, you should leverage highlight colors and account-specific messaging, such as "Past Due" or "Final Notice" as an occurrence ages within the collection process.

This helps patients clearly distinguish which balances are delinquent and which are current.

Challenge #3: Explaining how patient payments will be applied

By the same token, patients unable to pay the complete balance on their bill will want to know how partial payment will be applied to their overall balance. To avoid unnecessary patient calls to your business offices, ensure that this information is prominently displayed within your billing statement design.

Finally, it is important to note that a health system's ability to implement these design enhancements is dependent on the file output they select during their software conversion.

Choosing the best file output for your SBO conversion (PDF vs. FTF)

PDF Output – A PDF file format allows for a shorter conversion timeline. Therefore, this is the option most software providers will suggest.

However, any programming or dynamic design changes (like those mentioned above) are limited to the experience, capabilities, and workload capacity of the health system's internal resources.

FTF (Formatted Text File) Output

A FTF format can lengthen a health system's conversion timeline. In our experience, this option is least suggested by software providers.

However, this format allows the health system to customize their data file and maximize the effectiveness of their patient communication, by relying on the experience of their communication solution partner.

In addition, as health systems look to refine their patient engagement strategies post-conversion, the FTF output provides the flexibility

SBO - Single Billing Office

needed for future design optimization – ensuring they are able to meet the future communication needs of their organization.

The takeaway for RCM professionals

Life in healthcare revenue cycle isn't getting any easier. If you have the opportunity to redesign your patient statement, and develop a more complete patient engagement strategy, take advantage of it.

If you're issuing an RFP, demand more from your potential partners.

In today's Revenue Cycle marketplace, with limited resources and decreasing budgets, we believe choosing the correct partner as your patient engagement expert is more important today than it has ever been.

This partner should be able to communicate patient engagement trends, the latest in patient self-service technologies and how they will continue to optimize patient response post-conversion.

However, the way in which you decide to produce a data file (PDF or FTF) will have a significant impact on your success. This will either greatly enhance your ability to navigate and respond quickly to changing needs, or increase the work load and burden on your staff.

Choose wisely.

Chapter 4: How They Pay Is Half the Battle

Let Your Portal Do the Heavy Lifting

Every healthcare organization and medical office should have an online patient portal, but did you know that your portal is likely capable of more than you realize? Portal functions allow patients, physician offices, and health systems to share the same information and keep updated records.

Electronic health records (EHRs), appointment reminders, and payment capabilities are just the beginning of what you can do with portal technology. Patients of all ages are using portals to keep track of medication and personal health information, as well as account balances and payment history. A portal that meets all of a patient needs and desires is necessary to retain these "customers" in the healthcare marketplace.

Mobile Optimization

More than 57% of emails are opened on a phone or tablet. And almost 60% of all web traffic is now originating from a mobile device. If your portal is not mobile-friendly, your patients are not going to use it. Best practices have changed in the world of online portals, and a mobile-friendly site design is a top priority.

Mobile-friendly does not mean a website that you can simply see on a mobile device. It means a responsive site that is configured to work specifically within the confines of a smaller screen. Menus change and conform to the device screen; search capabilities are made "clickable" with the touch of a finger; and content is organized in a way that flows naturally with the scrolling behavior of mobile devices.

Patients should also be able to update communication preferences, receive medical records via email, and text messages for appointment reminders, as well as sync intuitively into their files and calendars. Consider this: when was the last time you asked for a reminder card? They are not needed when you can manage everything from your cell phone.

An Easy-to-Use Portal

Have you ever walked through the process of setting up a patient account on your portal? Did you get frustrated and want to give up? Patients expect portal account setup to be quick and helpful. If you are having issues, then your patients will have these hurdles, too, which is why they are probably not using it.

An easy-to-use portal must be simple, intuitive, with a few steps to register and little time involved to set up an account. One-step verification is necessary in making this happen. In addition, a clear set of instructions written for an uneducated audience (not for the portal developer) are must haves within your portal.

A level of user-based testing should also be incorporated to help validate how quickly and easily a patient can navigate through your portal, which will help reduce patient complaints and increase patient use.

Could Your Hospital Offer Remote Bill Payments?

According to Pew Research Center, nearly 80 percent of Americans own a smartphone; the number jumps to 85 percent for patients ages 18 to 64, and those 65 and older are gaining ground at nearly 50 percent[xvii]. At the other end of your patient base, 95 percent of millennials want to receive text messages about all aspects of care delivery—from front-office appointment reminders to back-office billing and payment options.

Much more than a talking and texting tool, the smartphone is a veritable life-management gadget. Taking advantage of countless apps, smartphone users can execute a variety of functions remotely. For example, users can control household appliances, monitor a security system, and even unlock car doors without being physically present. Moreover, anyone can make purchases and send payments using a connected smart device.

Apple® is a great example of a company that understands the needs and wants of its customers—and in turn, creates solutions to satisfy them. In reality, this should be the modus operandi of today's healthcare industry.

The patient is a healthcare consumer with very specific expectations. How hospitals, health systems, and providers respond to those expectations can determine whether they thrive financially in a very crowded market where patients have more choices than ever.

The good news is that the healthcare industry is no longer a laggard in the adoption of technology. The passage of ACA and HI-TECH have made it a business imperative for healthcare organizations to deploy electronic health records (EHRs) and other technology solutions to streamline administrative and clinical efficiencies. Even on the revenue cycle management front, vendors have developed technology to help healthcare providers increase revenues and reduce bad debt.

Convenient Payment Options and What Patients Expect from the Healthcare Facilities

If the financial world has shown us anything in recent years, it is the power of convenience. Buyers want options—secure options. From PayPal® to Bitcoin™, multiple methods of payment are expected in every industry.

According to a report on healthcare payment trends, online and e-wallets are on the rise as preferred payment channels. From 2013 to 2016, payments to providers through a health plan's website increased 527 percent, and payments from an online patient portal increased 139 percent[xviii]. Patients prefer omnichannel medical bill payment methods (58 percent voted for online options) and prefer to pay using credit and debit cards with a growing interest in mobile payment systems (also known as e-wallet systems), such as PayPal®, Apple Pay® and Android Pay®.

It's no surprise, then, that patients are expecting more convenience from their healthcare providers. In a financial climate where healthcare dollars are shrinking due to reduced reimbursements and increased bad debt, facilities should appeal to the desires of their consumers. Convenient and safe payment options are at the top of the list for most patients with nearly three in four patients indicating that online bill payment is their preferred channel.

Chapter 5: Leverage Intelligence at Every Touchpoint

Four steps to simplify account segmentation

Buying scores from a third-party provider that predict a patient's likelihood to pay or their prequalification for financial assistance is one of the most confusing and most underutilized RCM assets for most healthcare providers. Many providers feel hesitant to "waste" money on a score whose only application is to assign a patient to charity instead of bad debt. Others feel that buying propensity to pay scoring is also a useless investment, since their gut instinct is that the high propensity patients will pay anyway... so why pay for that data?

Unfortunately, many healthcare organizations remain stuck at this stage. Instead of using their data to work patient accounts more efficiently or engage patients more effectively within the revenue cycle, they remain stuck in analysis paralysis – not knowing where to start.

Here are four tips to help simplify the process and get started with account segmentation:

1. Start small

Typically, the word "segmentation" calls to mind large-scale, IT-intensive projects that require significant budget, time, and resources. In reality, segmenting patient accounts should be an iterative process.

Administrators should monitor results closely and make strategy changes as needed. With all of the options available, try starting with something that is easy to implement and does not require significant resources.

A few examples may include:
- Changing your intake script based on service area

- Making a letter or statement design changed based on a predictive model

- Adjusting patient communication channel (text, call, or IVR) or timing based on a patient's likelihood to make payment

A true segmentation strategy often starts with one small step. The best place to start is by determining one element in your process that, if improved, would make an impact on your bottom line.

2. Prioritize your metrics and find your quick wins

If you are new to segmenting patient accounts, focus your initial efforts on the metrics that correlate directly with your goals as a department or organization. After you've narrowed your focus, look for quick-win opportunities to influence these metrics.

Quick-wins can be defined as changes you can make to your current process that have the shortest implementation timeline and the most significant ROI potential.

The key is to not get stuck reviewing *all* of the data that is available to you. Prioritize your metrics and look for the easy wins that help your strategy gain momentum.

3. Establish a baseline

Before implementing any segmentation strategy, measure the metric you are trying to influence.

For example, if your priority is to reduce accounts receivables days and get patients to make payment sooner, what is the average number of days between a statement being mailed and a payment being received?

After you have an established baseline, and segmentation is in place, you can now measure the results of your strategy.

Have you improved patient response rates? Are patients making payment sooner?

Adjust your strategy accordingly.

4. Grow Over Time

Your segmentation strategy can grow based on what you learn along the way. Avoid being overwhelmed by starting small and staying focused on your unique goals.

But the key is to *start*.

An example of a more complex workflow that began with basic point of service area segmentation is shown below:

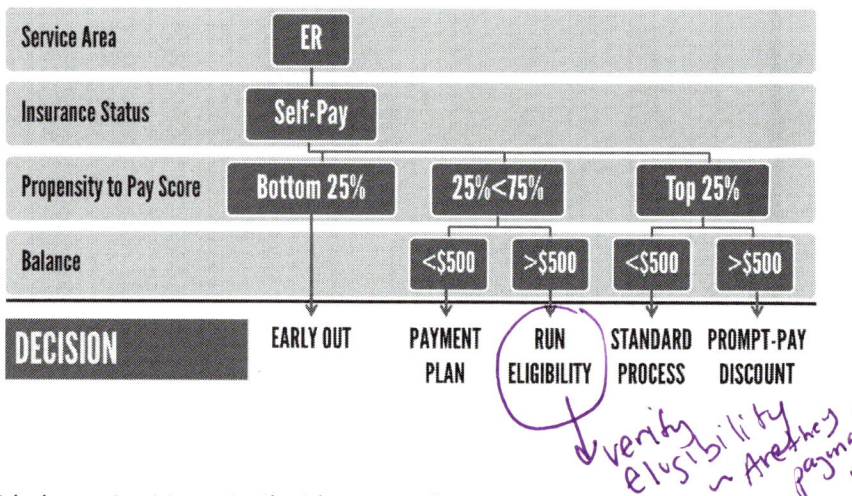

Service Area	ER			
Insurance Status	Self-Pay			
Propensity to Pay Score	Bottom 25%	25%<75%		Top 25%
Balance		<$500 / >$500	<$500 / >$500	
DECISION	EARLY OUT	PAYMENT PLAN	RUN ELIGIBILITY	STANDARD PROCESS	PROMPT-PAY DISCOUNT

[handwritten note: verify eligibility ~ Are they paying?]

It is important to note that how much your segmentation strategy grows is dependent on the automation capabilities of your organization, as well as the automation and customization capabilities of your vendor partners.

Want better results from predictive analytics? Try these proven strategies from other industries.

In comparison to other industries, healthcare revenue cycle is still relatively "young" when it comes to deploying big data and predictive models to improve business operations. Luckily, predictive analytics has been a staple in other industries for years. And many organizations in these industries are mastering the execution of predictive models.

Here are three tried and true applications of predictive modeling used in other industries, and how they can be used in healthcare revenue cycle.

1. Optimize patient payment arrangements to accelerate cashflow and account resolution.

In the credit card industry, predictive analytics are used to determine the Annual Percentage Rate (APR) of their cardholders.

Credit card companies have multiple predictive models in place that account for different factors about their cardholders, such as:

- their overall debt load
- their past history with the bank or lending institution
- the type of purchases they have made with credit cards

All of this data is then fed into a larger segmentation strategy to determine the cardholder's APR.

While hospitals can't leverage such a sliding scale because of 501(r) regulations, they *can* use similar models and scores to determine whether or not to offer prompt-pay discounts or automate payment plans.

2. Automate follow-up to at-risk populations to increase likelihood of response.

In the retail industry, how many times have you put an item in your online shopping cart only to close the browser and abandon the purchase altogether?

Some of the most innovative retail companies are using statistical models to get online shoppers to return to their site and complete the purchase. These statistical models predict whether or not a person will return to the site and make a purchase if he or she receives an automated reminder email.

Sometimes the email is a reminder that an item was left in their shopping cart, and other times it offers a discount for completing the purchase. The model dictates the offer that is presented in the email.

For hospitals using predictive models, sometimes patients fall into the "gray area" – do they qualify for presumptive charity? What about their likelihood to pay?

You may not have enough information to make a clear determination. However, if you know that a patient went to your online portal to pay or if you see their phone number in your IVR reporting, you can automate a follow-up phone call, text, or email to encourage them to finish their transaction if they did not make payment.

3. Create a sense of urgency by alternating communications based on the score.

The travel industry, particularly airlines, use a variety of predictive models based on third-party data to customize all offers and customer communications.

They account for factors such as:

- credit bureau data
- online activity
- past purchase behavior
- time of year

The model is used to both tailor the offer to prospective flyers and create urgency – leading to more booked flights for the airline.

Hospitals can adopt a similar strategy based on propensity to pay scoring. If you know a patient is likely to pay, as well as a seasonal time when they may have more disposable income (i.e. tax refund season), try creating a sense of urgency in your communications.

Example: Save 20% on your bill by making a payment before April 20, 2015.

Given the current RCM landscape, leveraging analytics can seem so overwhelming that it is too much to tackle right now with your current workload.

Front-End vs. Back-End Scoring & Segmentation: Which is best for your health system?

It's no secret today's healthcare business leaders are strapped for budget and staff resources.

And while most RCM leaders believe predictive scoring and account segmentation make it easier to work their patient accounts, there are differing opinions over *when* a score should be used.

Is it better to segment accounts at the point-of-service (Front-End) or at some point during the billing process (Back-End)?

The benefits of either approach

Before diving into a Front-End versus Back-End scoring discussion, it is important to point out that either approach can deliver significant returns to a healthcare organization. While there can be several advantages to scoring patient accounts, here are a few that are most critical:

1. Reducing cost to collect through automation
   - Reduced communications to patients

- Manage outsource vendors more efficiently

2. Adhering to policies & regulations (internal and external) and mission
- Identifying enough charity for 501 requirements
- Ensuring that your indigent population is being cared for financially

3. Public relations
- Enhancing the perception of your organization within your community

Now, the extent to which these benefits are realized will depend largely on the *execution* of your segmentation strategy, including *when* you decide to score accounts.

Front-End vs. Back-End Scoring: The two deciding factors

The timing of your segmentation comes down to two factors: (1) your organization's mission and (2) its tolerance or aggressiveness.

Mission

When Front-End segmentation makes sense...

If a healthcare system believes that their indigent population deserve free care (regardless of whether the patient would pay for given care or not), then it makes sense to utilize a charity score to identify financial assistance cases from the point of access. This approach moves as many qualified patients as possible into their charity program.

Although this approach was not strongly embraced over 10 years ago, we will see more of it, especially with the government now mandating charity care. Also, point-of-service scoring can help to identify potential Medicaid enrollees, which can lead to additional reimbursement.

When Back End segmentation makes sense...

If a healthcare system is simply scoring to avoid negative public relations and identifying charity cases before sending them to a bad debt agency, then scoring after billing makes sense. However, a majority of the benefits of scoring are lost in this scenario.

Tolerance / Aggressiveness

Some patients will actually pay their bills, after the first or second statement, even though they would score into a charity program.

This leads many to the conclusion that scoring after billing makes more sense. However, that's not always the case.

In this scenario, an analysis should be leveraged to validate this approach. This analysis should compare the overall cost of billing versus what is collected. While scoring at the front end may move "self-pay payers" from paying their bill into charity care, does the cost of a score and the lost collection dollars outweigh the cost of collecting those balances?

Organizations utilizing a score on the front end to drive segmentation and collections workflows are better positioned to move the needle by:

1. Accelerating cash flow. Prioritizing accounts earlier in the revenue cycle and refocusing the efforts of staff can influence patients to make payment faster.

2. Reducing cost to collect. Along these same lines, earlier segmentation allows organizations to take action sooner, so they can:

- Insource accounts that are "easy" to collect and reduce contingency fees
- Reduce and optimize their patient balance communications
- Reduce inbound patient calls to their business office

There are benefits to scoring regardless of the approach that is taken. However, implementing a strategy that aligns with your organization's business objectives requires understanding both the mission of your healthcare system, and how proactive you want to be within your segmentation and AR collection efforts.

Let's drill deeper into front-end vs. back-end scoring.

Front-end scoring

The drawback
It can be argued that using a front-end scoring process may cause hospitals to lose potential revenue from individuals. For instance, patients could be scored as charity eligible or unable to make payment—when in reality, they have other methods to acquire the funds needed, methods that a scoring model may not have the capability to address.

The benefits
The advantage to front-end scoring is validation of the collectability of an organization's AR as quickly after service as possible. Organizations know what they can expect when it comes to cash collections and can draft a hospital charity policy to insure those who are unable to pay due to income and/or prior history are categorized as charity care.

Also, front-end scoring is helpful from a public relations standpoint and aids in 501 (c)(3) compliance – making reasonable efforts to determine whether an individual is eligible for assistance.

This process can significantly reduce the amount of effort required on the back end. Touching all accounts on the front end is a frightening proposition for many hospitals because it appears to add considerable expense up front.

A more proactive and financially conservative approach to front-end scoring would be to score only the straight self-pay or uninsured accounts.

Additional considerations for front-end scoring
Commercial contracts. Even though a patient may prove to be charity eligible based on the score the hospital may be contractually obligated to complete certain collection efforts prior to charity consideration. This further substantiates the reason to use the front-end scoring approach on the uninsured accounts only.

Charity policy. The other key to front-end scoring is to clearly illustrate in the hospitals charity policy how accounts are considered in the process. Implementing a front-end process may also require internal process and staffing changes that a hospital may be apprehensive to adopt due to other competing priorities.

Back-end scoring

The benefits
Back-end scoring can mean a number of things, but in this case consider back-end to be prior to bad debt placement.

The advantage to back-end scoring is that it will come at a significantly lower price than front-end scoring, based on volume.

Also, scoring accounts prior to bad debt placement is definitely better than not scoring at all from a public relations standpoint and can also aid in 501 (c)(3) compliance as mentioned in the front-end scoring section.

The drawback
What this approach does not consider is the amount of work required to resolve accounts later in the process – chasing accounts which, if scored, would require no work effort. After accounts cycle through the AR process, many will drop out due to payment resolution, no balance due after insurance, or for other various reasons.

Additional considerations for back-end scoring
Self-pay and uninsured patients. At the back end, it makes sense to consider your self-pay/uninsured population along with the patients

covered by insurance – providing one last attempt to correctly categorize accounts prior to bad debt placement.

In a situation where a front-end scoring process is already in place for self-pay/uninsured patients, an additional back-end scoring process for insured patients makes sense from a compliance perspective (with the Affordable Care Act).

The important piece to consider when implementing either or both approaches is insuring facility processes and policies clearly illustrate how accounts are processed and considered within the individual scoring model selected. When in doubt discuss plans with your auditors to insure everything is in order.

Chapter 6: Ensure Compliance and Security

501(r): What You Need to Know
Summary of 501(r)
As part of the Affordable Care Act, the IRS added four new requirements for hospitals to continue to qualify as tax-exempt entities:

- Community Health Needs Assessments completed
- Written and Financial Assistance Policies that are easy to find, request, receive, and understand
- A policy that limits charges for indigent populations
- Compliance with guidelines for billing and collections on individuals that may qualify for financial assistance

This measure is intended to hold hospitals accountable for meeting their local community's financial needs in order to justify their tax-exempt status. This measure took effect in January 2011; however, the deadline for compliance has not yet been set. In June 2012, more detailed requirements for 501(r)(4)(5)(6) were published in the federal register.

- 501(r)(4) deals with a hospital's Financial Assistance Policy requirements
- 501(r)(5) addresses setting limits on charges and how charges are calculated
- 501(r)(6) ensures that all reasonable efforts are made to determine whether or not a patient is eligible for charity before engaging in Extraordinary Collections Actions

Financial Assistance Policy
How a hospital provides financial assistance for the local community is one of the key foundational pieces of 501(r). Section 4 lists several

criteria that must be included in a hospital's Financial Assistance Policy to be compliant. A high-level overview is shown in the chart below.

Component	Requirement
Plain-language version	If the Financial Assistance policy contains legal language or business contract language, it will need to be modified to a ninth grade reading level.
Policy available in other languages	If more than 10 percent of the residents of within the community surrounding a hospital facility speak a language other than English, the Financial Assistance Policy must be available in that language.
Include ECA's	Any Extraordinary Collections Actions a hospital may undertake in an effort to collect must be included in the Financial Assistance Policy.
Widely available	The Financial Assistance Policy should be available in print or digital format, available on request.
Publicized	References on how to find a copy of the Financial Assistance Policy (if not already included) must be on every applicable patient communication.

Reasonable Efforts on Screening

Section 6 of the 501(r) Guidelines states that for hospitals to be compliant, they must make "reasonable" efforts to determine whether or not someone is eligible for charity before engaging in any extraordinary collections activities. What this means is that if a hospital believes there is a possibility of a patient qualifying for charity, several communications must be sent throughout the revenue cycle. The chart below outlines high-level requirements.

Timing	Requirement
Prior to discharge	Provide a copy of the Financial Assistance Policy and Charity Application to each patient or guarantor
Notification Period	From time of service to 120 days post discharge, the Financial Assistance Policy must be included with all bills sent (minimum requirement of at least three bills). Additionally, written notice of ECA's that may be taken must be provided.
Application Period	From the first bill mailed date to 240 days post discharge, the patient is eligible to apply for assistance

The tricky part is the relationship between the notification period and the application period. Based on present guidelines, there is the potential for collection actions to be taken between 120 and 240 days. This can be problematic if collections actions are underway, and the patient applies for assistance. In that situation, the hospital is responsible for reversing all of those collection actions.

Changing the process at intake is an immense undertaking

Depending on where the patient is admitted, a hospital may be missing information needed to help determine if the patient may be eligible for financial assistance. An important point to remember: under the new guidelines, hospitals **cannot** deny financial assistance for missing or incomplete information from the patient. Even an incomplete charity application is not a basis for refusing aid.

Does this mean that hospitals will need to change their point-of-service process to obtain more accurate demographic or financial information? While that is one valid option, it can take significant time, money, and resources to achieve the desired results. Additionally, changing processes to gather enough information to do a complete charity screening is likely to take a back seat to larger initiatives like ICD-10 or a systems conversion.

Implementing a scoring solution that works within an existing process is the best option. Scoring solutions utilize patient information you have received, match that information against third party external databases in real time, and then screen for:

- Identity verification (fraud detection)
- Presumptive charity (likelihood to qualify for financial assistance based upon your hospital's policy)
- Propensity to pay (likelihood to pay outstanding balance)

How do you determine eligibility with existing processes?

Many forward-thinking hospitals and medical centers are starting to use external vendors to validate and supplement incomplete patient information, to better determine eligibility for financial assistance. Presumptive charity scoring takes a guarantor's information and matches it against public data sources to give hospitals a more comprehensive view of a patient's financial situation. The scoring process can occur within existing registration or statement processing and requires little IT resource requirements or disruption to a hospitals existing patient access process flows. Typically, the implementation for integrating predictive scores in a hospital's current process takes approximately 30 days and can cost a fraction of a traditional database solution.

An in-line scoring solution allows revenue cycle administrators to set business rules on who to score and how to process those accounts based on the score. This significantly reduces the need for manual work and can free up existing employees to focus their time on working patient accounts and less time on manual review, which may provide cost savings by reducing statement mailing costs. A solution such as this can be implemented with little or no change to existing workflows.

Summary

The two most significant changes from 501(r) that will impact hospitals are:

- Making the Financial Assistance Policy easy-to-read, accessible, and communicated with every patient communication
- Ensuring adequate and thorough screening of all patients for financial assistance eligibility

The level of effort required to modify the Financial Assistance Policy is small compared to any process changes that may be required in order to get all the information needed to make a determination on whether or not a patient qualifies for financial assistance. In the latter scenario, it is highly recommended that hospitals use charity scoring solutions to fill in the gaps.

Complying with 501(r) regulations is a challenging task for hospitals. While the effort to modify existing Financial Assistance Policies is not difficult, ensuring that patients receive the policy consistently while also implementing a screening process that is auditable without disruption of existing processes can be a daunting task. By implementing an analytic charity scoring solution with an integrated communication and audit plan, hospitals can achieve compliance with the new regulations and keep workflow processes virtually unchanged while improving patient satisfaction.

Is your healthcare organization ready for EMV?

Today, if a credit or debit card is swiped to make a payment, the bank that issued the card is liable for the costs of any fraudulent transactions – but that is about to change.

On October 1, 2015, any merchant processing "swipe and sign" card transactions must also be able to process Europay, Mastercard, and Visa (EMV) transactions – or be forced to accept the financial responsibility of counterfeit card losses.

So, what is EMV? How do EMV transactions work? And how does a healthcare organization prepare for the "liability shift?"

What is EMV?

EMV is the global standard for chip card technology, and the devices or terminals used to authenticate chip card transactions.

These new cards have a microchip embedded in the plastic and are referred to as chip cards or EMV cards. Instead of reading a magnetic stripe, EMV terminals read the microchip embedded in the card – helping protect cardholder information and fight card fraud.

How does an EMV card work?
Instead of a traditional "swipe & sign" transaction, EMV transactions use a "dip" method.

This means a consumer "dips" his or her card into the payment terminal and keeps it there during the payment process. Once the transaction is approved, the cardholder confirms the amount by either entering a four-digit PIN number or providing their signature on the terminal – depending on what is required by the card issuer.

However, it is important to note that chip cards will not put an end to swipe & sign transactions.

EMV cards still have the magnetic stripe on the back of the card, which means merchants do not *have* to invest in devices that process EMV transactions.

But, not obtaining the equipment necessary for EMV transactions could mean greater financial liability for merchants.

What does it mean for healthcare providers?
The first step in creating a solution is to understand the problem. Cyber attacks on healthcare organization are on the rise, increasing 320 percent from 2015 to 2016 according to a 2017 Redspin report[xix]. To address the elevated threat, healthcare organization need solutions that:

- Increase payment card security
- Remain compliant with PCI requirements
- Reduce the scope of the card data environment
- Segment residual card data onto a network separate from clinical and EHR data

Payment Card Industry Data Security Standards Compliance (PCI-DSS) is the generally recognized set of security standards that organizations must adhere to if they accept credit card payments. The basic policies include controlling card data access, monitoring and tracking card data, and addressing information security within the organization with third party vendors. Compliance with PCI-DSS requires ongoing attention and vigilance.

Security Layers to Implement

To ensure security, a layered approach is recommended – above and beyond the PCI-DSS standards. Additional tools are available to reduce fraud and discourage hacking.

These include:

EMV®(Europay, Mastercard, and Visa) are the chip-enabled cards that have become the new standard. It's estimated[xx] that in 2017, 98% of cards issues in the U.S. will be chip cards. EMV cards offer a higher level of security than traditional magnetic strip because the chip enables card authentication to verify that the card is legitimate. Business receiving transactions have moved toward updating their card readers to work with chip cards, and healthcare organizations are also adopting these practices.

Encryption is used to scramble the card data into a different form – cipher text – while it travels through the POS system and over the payment network. The cipher text cannot be easily read except with the authorized "decoder".

Tokenization removes the card data from the provider's environment which protects the card data at rest. The card number is replaced by a randomly generated token, which makes it useless to thieves, but allows it to remain "on file" in a safe way. The token is specific to the merchant or business, so it doesn't carry any information if intercepted by an outside source.

A comprehensive approach to data security, including and especially in the payment process, is critical to keeping patient data secure during their healthcare interactions.

Final Thoughts

The only constant in the healthcare industry is change.

Since the 2010 passage of the Affordable Care Act (ACA), healthcare has changed dramatically. As a result, conventional approaches to achieving clinical and financial excellence are shifting. Hospitals and providers have a critical business imperative to implement effective operational strategies to keep up with healthcare's regulatory, technological, clinical, and financial changes while maintaining profitability. From new methods of care delivery and the redefined role of the healthcare provider to evolving reimbursement models and big data, the impacts are great. Healthcare organizations will do well to seek out technology innovation partners to help them prepare for these changes with the information, guidance, and solutions needed to thrive in an everchanging and competitive market.

Industry experts believe that in the coming years technological developments in the areas of database infrastructure, decision support platforms, and mobile communication devices will enable providers and payers to thwart disease progression and reduce unnecessary hospital admissions and emergency room visits, which are the foundation of population health management.

Healthcare organizations must be forward-thinking and willing to adapt to change, or else they will be left behind. Hospitals and providers seeking to stand out from the crowd would do well to enlist the services of experienced industry partners that can help them deploy technology and processes that will enable them to respond agilely to current and future changes in healthcare.

About the Authors

Marty Callahan brings more than 25 years of demonstrated leadership and business development experience in healthcare and consumer finance services to RevSpring. His extensive knowledge of predictive analytics, data management, decisioning systems, and business rules automation helps healthcare organizations keep up with changing industry trends.

Casey Williams has over 15 years of experience in developing customized patient communications and payment solutions for over 100 healthcare revenue cycle clients. His knowledge of patient engagement strategies, including self-service optimization, has made him a go-to speaker and presenter for HFMA, Healthcare Finance Institute, and Litmos Healthcare Division (formerly Bridgefront) to name a few.

April Elliott Wilson has a long history of measuring and optimizing meaningful communication for top brands. April is the Vice President of Analytics and Marketing at RevSpring, where she has co-engineered the Intelligent Workflow Solutions program. She has served on the Board of Directors for the Web Analytics Association and has also taught MBA courses for Southern Methodist University, Otterbein University, and Stanford.

RevSpring is a leading provider of consumer communications and billing solutions that maximize revenue opportunities for collections agencies, credit grantors, and healthcare providers. Since 1981, RevSpring has built the industry's most comprehensive and impactful suite of consumer engagement, communications, and payment pathways that is backed by consumer behavior analysis, propensity-to-pay scoring, intelligent design, and user experience best practices. To learn more, visit www.revspringinc.com or contact learnmore@revspringinc.com.

References

[i] Patient Loyalty: It's up for grabs. Accenture Strategy. https://www.accenture.com/t20160322T034105Z__w__/ca-en/_acnmedia/Accenture/Conversion-Assets/DotCom/Documents/Global/PDF/Strategy_7/Accenture-Strategy-Patient-Engagement-Consumer-Loyalty.pdf

[ii] RevSpring proprietary research; front-end contact study 2017.

[iii] Americans Check their Phones 80 times a day: study. https://nypost.com/2017/11/08/americans-check-their-phones-80-times-a-day-study/

[iv] Setting Goals: Who, Why, How? Citation: Turkay, S. (2014). Setting Goals: Who, Why, How?. Manuscript.

[v] The Small-Area Hypothesis: Effects of Progress Monitoring on Goal Adherence Author(s): Minjung Koo and Ayelet Fishbach Reviewed work(s): Source: Journal of Consumer Research, (-Not available-), p. 000 Published by: The University of Chicago Press Stable URL: http://www.jstor.org/stable/10.1086/663827

[vi] How To Implement Incentives That Actually Work. https://www.forbes.com/sites/forbescoachescouncil/2017/04/24/how-to-implement-incentives-that-actually-work/

[vii] Pros and Cons of Monetary Incentives Compensation Bridget Miller Wednesday - January 14, 2015. https://hrdailyadvisor.blr.com/2015/01/14/pros-and-cons-of-monetary-incentives/

[viii] How One Hospital Embraced Patient Satisfaction Transparency. https://www.healthcatalyst.com/success_stories/transparency-in-healthcare

[ix] Working Families at Risk: Coverage, Access, Cost and Worries. https://www.kff.org/uninsured/working-families-at-risk-coverage-access-cost/

[x] Mad*Pow 2016 Study:
https://static1.squarespace.com/static/5715100cf8baf3c79d443859/t/5730e1c4f699bbe627603424/1462821330491/DesignChallenge_ResearchReport.pdf

[xi] Hospital revenue cycle operations: Opportunities created by the ACA.
http://healthcare.mckinsey.com/sites/default/files/MCK_Hosp_Full_Issue.pdf

[xii] Surviving the Deductible Reset in 2012: How to Collect Deductibles and Improve Self Pay Collections. Sara M. Larch, MSHA, FACMPE January 9th, 2012. http://gettingpaid.kareo.com/gettingpaid/2012/01/lets-collect-deductibles-in-2012-tips-for-improving-self-pay-collections/

[xiii] US Census Projections

[xiv] http://www.pewinternet.org/2017/05/17/barriers-to-adoption-and-attitudes-towards-technology/

[xv] http://www.pewinternet.org/2017/05/17/barriers-to-adoption-and-attitudes-towards-technology/

[xvi] Patient Financial Responsibility Increased 11% in 2017: A Study. https://www.revcycleintelligence.com/news/patient-financial-responsibility-increased-11-in-2017

[xvii] http://www.pewresearch.org/fact-tank/2017/06/28/10-facts-about-smartphones/

[xviii] http://healthpromedical.com/wp-content/uploads/2017/11/Trends_in_Healthcare_Payments_Annual_Report_2016.pdf

[xix] https://healthitsecurity.com/news/healthcare-cybersecurity-attacks-rise-320-from-2015-to-2016

[xx] https://www.creditcards.com/credit-card-news/emv-chip-cards-arrive-poll.php

Made in the USA
Columbia, SC
29 June 2020